MW01291745

MEDITERRANEAN DIET FOR BEGINNERS

A Beginner's Guide to the Mediterranean Diet with Recipes and Meal Plans

Text Copyright © Light Bulb Publishing

All rights reserved. No part of this guide may be reproduced in any form without permission in writing from the publisher except in the case of brief quotations embodied in critical articles or reviews.

Legal & Disclaimer

The information contained in this book and its contents is not designed to replace or take the place of any form of medical or professional advice; and is not meant to replace the need for independent medical, financial, legal or other professional advice or services, as may be required. The content and information in this book has been provided for educational and entertainment purposes only.

The content and information contained in this book has been compiled from sources deemed reliable, and it is accurate to the best of the Author's knowledge, information, and belief. However, the Author cannot guarantee its accuracy and validity and cannot be held liable for any errors and/or omissions. Further, changes are periodically made to this book as and when needed. Where appropriate and/or necessary, you must consult a professional (including but not limited to your doctor, attorney, financial advisor or such other professional advisor) before using any of the suggested remedies, techniques, or information in this book.

Upon using the contents and information contained in this book, you agree to hold harmless the Author from and against any damages, costs, and expenses, including any legal fees potentially resulting from the application of any of the information provided by this book. This disclaimer applies to any loss, damages or injury caused by the use and application, whether directly or indirectly, of any advice or information presented, whether for breach of contract, tort, negligence, personal injury, criminal intent, or under any other cause of action.

You agree to accept all risks of using the information presented in this book.

You agree that by continuing to read this book, where appropriate and/or necessary, you shall consult a professional (including but not limited to your doctor, attorney, or financial advisor or such other advisor as needed) before using any of the suggested remedies, techniques, or information in this book.

Table of Contents

Introduction

What is the Mediterranean diet?

The name "Mediterranean diet" has an antique ring to it – it suggests that we are talking about something that was set in place millennia ago. In a sense that is true, but not necessarily in the way we imagine it. It is not something that Roman emperors were eating, nor is it something that Ancient Greece was famous for. The Mediterranean diet is relatively new. It's based on the diet prevalent among the people of Greece, Southern Italy and Spain in the 1960s. That is a wide territory and the foods eaten in those areas differ. What brought them all together into what we now call the Mediterranean diet are the features that they all share:

- High intake of unsaturated healthy fats

- Little to no processed or refined foods

- Fruits eaten daily

- Non-starchy vegetables eaten with almost every meal

- Limited amount of poultry and especially red meat

- Fish and seafood as the main protein source

- Herbs and seasonings instead of salt

- Red wine (this one is optional, and should be, by some estimates, limited to 14 units[1] per week)

---

[1] Alcohol unit is a way to determine how strong your drink is. For usual red wine (13% alcohol), there are around 3 units per big glass (250ml). On a weekly scale, that would mean you can have a bottle and a half (1,25l) of wine without any significant health risks.

This diet became popular in the United States because of the realization that people from the Mediterranean area tend to live longer and have a much smaller risk of cardiovascular disease. There is also a very low obesity rate in that part of the world, and most of the people stay active and agile long after they retire.

There are five so called *blue zones* – areas throughout the world where people have the longest life expectancies and a very low risk of diseases prevalent in the modern West, such as type II diabetes and cancer. Two of those five zones are in the Mediterranean – the Italian island of Sardinia, and Ikaria, an isolated island in Greece. Not only do people there tend to live longer on average, they also often live to be 100 years old.

Some believe their longevity and health are the result of low stress levels. Some think it is the food that holds the key to their vitality. Some think it's just fortunate genetics. Due to the multitude of factors involved it is difficult to determine what exactly is the secret of their success.

I am far from saying that diet alone can be the cause of longevity and superior health; a low-stress lifestyle in a tight-knit community plays a role as well. But the diet people in the Mediterranean eat also contributes to their well-being. We will get into the specifics of eating in the chapters that follow, but it's also worth mentioning that people in the Mediterranean eat in a different way than what we might expect.

Unlike your typical western family that maybe gets together for dinner, people from Italy, Greece and Spain eat most of their meals together as a family. There is not a whole lot of snacking in between meals, and every meal is basically a mini party. Most meals are cooked, and they are never junk food.

They also take more time to eat, which means two things: stress relief in conversation with people close to you, and eating slowly to give yourself a chance to feel full, which usually prevents overeating. It may not seem like much, but the feeling of closeness that comes from this practice can enrich our lives and make us more relaxed.

Now that we know what the Mediterranean diet is, let's see who it is for and why you should consider giving it a go.

What the Mediterranean Diet is Not

While the Mediterranean diet is not that complicated to wrap your mind around, it is quite easy to trick ourselves into thinking that we are following the Mediterranean diet when we, in fact, are not. That is because people still have many misconceptions about what the Mediterranean diet is and is not.

Changing the way we eat (especially from a non-restrictive kind where we are constantly overfed) can be a traumatic experience for our psyches, so we expect rationalizations and excuses. Here are some of the facts to keep in mind when thinking about the Mediterranean diet:

1. Pizza and pasta are not Mediterranean dishes.

    Yes, there is nothing more quintessentially Italian than pizza, and yes, pasta comes to mind next when you think of this lovely country, but unfortunately, these dishes are not staple foods of the Mediterranean diet. You can still eat both of those foods from time to time, but you should consider them treat meals. It's not that pizza and pasta are all bad, but they are too high in calories. They also contain carbohydrates that are less complex than those in other Mediterranean dishes.

2. Canned fruit does not count as a healthy snack.

The Mediterranean diet is based largely on vegetables and fruits. Their high nutritional value, abundance of fiber and low calorie count all make them the perfect choice for anybody trying to stay healthy and lean. However, it is important to keep in mind that fresh fruit and their canned counterpart are very different.

Canned fruit is higher in calories due to added sugar and its nutrients are depleted from processing. There is also a risk of developing botulism, a rare, but in some cases fatal illness, if the fruit is not canned properly.

Of course not all manufacturers are the same, and some use less sugary syrup than others, so if you are dead set on eating canned fruit once in a while, I won't stop you, but be sure to read the labels, avoid damaged cans, and opt for fresh fruit whenever you can.

3. Snacking occasionally is okay, but keep yourself accountable.

We have already established that following a new eating plan can be challenging. This is especially true for someone who was used to eating everything in sight. We adapt in different ways, so it's understandable that some people will have an easier time adhering to a diet if they make a clean-cut change from an unhealthy to a healthy way of eating.

However, most people lean toward the other end of the spectrum. We need something to look forward to, like a treat meal (I don't like the term cheat meal, as it is not cheating if you planned it) to celebrate an important milestone, or to keep us sane when dieting becomes too hard.

Now, this slippery slope can be dangerous. "Just this once" turns into "just twice a week," and excuses for snacking become easier and easier to find. That is why it is important to keep yourself accountable, just like with any other diet.

There are many ways to do this:

- Start the Mediterranean diet with a friend or partner, so you can help each other through difficult parts.

- Keep a food journal to give you a clearer picture of how often you are slipping.

- Get a calorie tracking app on your smartphone. You can even set an alarm for your treat meal.

- If you want, you can post your progress on social media. Not only will you have the whole community to hold you accountable, but you might help somebody else make the right choice, or avoid some of the mistakes you have made.

4. Too much of a good thing is still a bad thing.

    This point drives the previous message home. Eating too much healthy food is still going to make you gain weight. The Mediterranean diet is designed to make it difficult to overeat (thanks to the high fiber content and relying on vegetables and fruits for many of your daily calories).

    On the other hand, fats (healthy and unhealthy alike) contain more calories per gram than carbohydrates or protein (a gram of fat contains approximately 9kcal, and a gram of carbs or protein amounts to only 4kcal). That is why it is important to keep in mind how calorie dense healthy fats are when you snack on nuts.

    It is incredibly easy to eat more than just a handful of peanuts when you're hungry, and the fact that nuts are healthy can be enough to trick us into thinking that we are eating the right way, when in fact we are consuming more than we need. I am not saying you need to count every cashew every time you snack, but be aware of the calorie content of healthy fats and be sure to stop at a handful.

Who is the Mediterranean Diet for?

The word "diet" has gotten a bad name over the years, and it's not my favorite word either, but not for the reasons you might think. The phrase "on a diet" implies that at some point in the future, you are going to be off it.

Any way of eating that is too restrictive or dangerous to follow for a prolonged period of time is not a diet you want to be on. (This does not include diets prescribed for medical reasons.)

The Keto diet has its benefits, but it may not be the best choice for you if you can't picture yourself abstaining from carbs for the rest of your days. Intermittent fasting works, sure, but difficulties will arise with changes in your daily schedule. Just imagine changing your job, moving to a different place, or having kids, and you will understand that sticking to your six-hour eating window will not be a piece of cake.

One of the best things about the Mediterranean diet is that it carries virtually no risk and it doesn't disrupt your eating schedule. Take it from the people living around the Mediterranean – do you think they care for timing each meal perfectly? Of course not. In other words, this diet will do wonders for you if you want it to, and if you do it right.

The health and fitness industry is commonly overwhelmed with new diet trends and fads, and people who give unrealistic promises. The question of all questions is, "How do I lose weight?" Ignore the "newly-found mechanism" that helps you burn fat faster, detox, cleanse, etc., and remember that eating fewer calories than you expend is the only way to lose weight.

There is no way to hack your metabolism, no secret formula to unlock your fat-burning potential, and especially no magic pill that will help you lose weight without putting in the work.

The Mediterranean diet has no magical properties. Put simply, you are eating less than you spend (usually), and you lose weight more easily because you don't constantly feel hungry due to the high fiber and protein intake. Also, your food cravings are much easier to control once you get rid of the sugary foods. This eliminates the insulin rollercoaster which is responsible for sugar crashes which is when you feel the most hungry and prone to reaching for snacks.

The only caveat is the same as any other diet – allergies. If you suffer from gluten intolerance, get rid of the foods that contain gluten. Lactose intolerance is easily avoidable by abstaining from dairy. Hypersensitivity to any other ingredient is manageable, if you just modify the diet accordingly.

The one allergy that is significant with the Mediterranean diet is a seafood allergy. As seafood makes up most of your protein intake, you might find it cumbersome to hit your daily protein goals. Protein is paramount when it comes to building muscle and preserving muscle mass when you are losing weight, so you can see why having enough of it is important.

On the other hand, there is no need to throw in the towel just yet. There are plenty of other ways to eat this way and still manage to get enough protein to promote muscle growth and weight loss. Protein is made up of amino acids. There are 22 in total, but nine of them are known as essential amino acids because our bodies can't produce them on their own. Complete proteins contain all nine of them.

The Mediterranean diet is more than just seafood and olive oil. Some grains, such as chickpeas and quinoa, are complete proteins, even though their biological values (the ability of our body to absorb and use it) is not the same as those of eggs or meat. Scientists have also discovered that some foods are higher in certain amino acids. So, if you pay some attention to pairing your legumes with grains (you don't even have to eat them in the same meal), you can get enough complete protein.

The Mediterranean diet can work for almost everybody and there are no conditions that prohibit a person from eating this way. Pay attention to your body, and consult a nutritionist if you have any allergies. If you are allergic to shellfish or seafood in general, there are many different ways to maintain this diet and reap the benefits from it. Now that we have answered what the Mediterranean diet is and who can follow it, let's discuss what makes this diet better than others.

What are the Health Benefits?

People who are looking for a new diet are usually looking for one thing and one thing alone: a way to lose weight. There is nothing wrong with wanting to fit into that dress from five years ago or get rid of the flabby belly your wife has been teasing you about. But there is a bigger picture here, and being slim is only a brushstroke on that canvas.

I am talking about your general health, longevity and improved quality of life. We have already determined that any eating plan will make you lose weight if it involves caloric deficit (eating less than you spend). A calorie is a calorie, whether it comes from a fast food joint or your grandmother's garden. You will lose weight eating a slice of pizza and a piece of cake a day, but imagine how that eating regimen would make you feel, and more importantly, what it would do to your body in the long run.

This diet is so much more than your cookie-cutter "lose some weight before the summer comes" tool. It is designed to make you lose fat, but also to help you feel better, have more energy, sleep better and be happier overall. Following the Mediterranean diet can bring about a world of change, so let's dive in and talk about what will happen to your body if you give it a go:

- You will lose weight.

  - The Mediterranean diet is rich in vegetables that contain very few calories. Also, as the majority of the carbohydrates you eat on this diet are complex, you will have more energy and no insulin crashes that occur when you eat simple carbs (sugars). The high fiber content of these foods will also keep you full longer, so you won't be so tempted to snack. Even the protein sources you rely on are far less calorically expensive than red meat.

- Your heart's health will improve.

  - This is one of the most well-known benefits of the Mediterranean diet. Likely thanks to the amount of healthy omega-3 fatty acids you consume while eating this way, the risk of heart attack, coronary disease and stroke decreases significantly. Another reason for this may be that the Mediterranean diet doesn't include much salt, which makes it one of the most heart friendly diets out there. Your triglycerides, cholesterol and blood pressure will likely improve if you follow the Mediterranean diet.

- Your blood sugar levels will be more stable.

  - Thanks to the abundance of complex carbohydrates and fiber you consume when you eat this way, you are far less likely to suffer from type II diabetes when you follow the Mediterranean diet. The prevalence of this disease is increasing, and it is closely linked to refined carbs and chronic stress, which are both absent from the Mediterranean lifestyle.

  - I know it can be difficult to abstain from eating anything sweet, but there is a way around that. Even though fruit doesn't sound like the tastiest of treats when you are craving ice cream, it can be a powerful tool in fighting off worse temptations. The longer you stay on this diet, the more apt at anticipating food cravings you will become. A strawberry now can stop a craving for an entire chocolate bar later.

- Your bone density will improve.

  - Our bones become more frail and brittle as we mature, and that is even more true for women. This is a result of a gradual decrease in bone density, especially in people who live a sedentary lifestyle. If you decide to follow an exercise program based on resistance training, you can diminish the risk of bone density loss even further.

— If you follow the Mediterranean diet, you can counteract this. It's still not certain what part of the Mediterranean diet makes a difference when it comes to bone health, but my guess is olive oil, as there is some evidence that consuming it increases the proliferation and maturation of bone cells.

• Your brain will work better in the long run.

— As we get older, our brains get older too. The health and function of your brain partly depends on the nutrients it receives. What fuels our brain is a complex subject, but the healthier your blood vessels are, the more nutrients your brain gets and the longer it keeps its cognitive potential. Imagine that those nutrients are traveling in trucks, and our blood vessels are highways. The less traffic there is, the more efficient the supply will be.

— Some studies suggest that people who adhere more closely to the Mediterranean diet have a lower risk of cognitive decline, and even Alzheimer's. That is partly due to the clear path for the blood to carry nutrients around. Another potential reason is that fatty acids (especially omega-3s) promote brain health, and following the Mediterranean diet is a sure way to get more than enough of them.

- You can prevent certain types of cancer.

  – Thanks to the high amounts of fiber, vitamins and antioxidants found in the fruits and vegetables that people on the Mediterranean diet eat, the risk of those people developing colorectal or breast cancer drops significantly. Given that colorectal cancer is one of the most common types of cancer among men, and breast cancer is the most common type of cancer among women, you can see why following this diet can be not only a positive change in a person's life, but a lifesaving choice as well.

  – Olive oil helps here as well. Women who adhere to the Mediterranean diet have up to 62% lower risk of cancer than women who follow a low-fat diet. Olive oil contains unsaturated fats, which means that it can bind other molecules to itself. Those things can be metabolites or other things that can be harmful for our bodies.

These are only some of the benefits of the Mediterranean diet. In addition to protecting your health, promoting gut health, keeping your brain young and agile, improving your bone density, preventing some of the most vicious of diseases, and helping with weight loss, this diet can also improve your mood, make you feel more energetic and even ease depression. In the chapters that follow, we will go over some of the basics of this way of eating.

Getting Started

Any lifestyle change can be a challenge. We don't like change, especially when it affects big chunks of our daily routine. That's why it's so easy to find excuses and reasons not to do it. There are quite a few misconceptions about the Mediterranean diet as well; the two I hear the most are:

- it's too expensive and

- it takes too much time to cook that way.

If you do it the right way, and the smart way, neither of those things have to be true. Apart from seafood (and only in some parts of the world), the groceries that make up most of the Mediterranean diet are easy to find. You can hunt for sales or buy in bulk to save money. It doesn't have to be too time consuming either. In fact, most of the Mediterranean meals are raw, and you can prepare them in minutes. If you want to cook as well, using Sunday mornings for meal preparation can set you up for the entire week. Remember, there is always a way, so there is no need to make excuses.

Another thing I love about this diet is that there are no side effects (if you don't have any allergies, and please check that before starting any diet), nor does it require a specific adaptation period. What that means is that you don't have to ease yourself into it. You have probably eaten most of these foods before, now it's just more of the good stuff.

Some other diets come with this sort of caveat. For example, people who start the Keto diet sometimes suffer from "Keto flu," with lovely side effects such as nausea, vomiting, diarrhea, fever and dizziness. That inconvenience can make people reluctant to even try a diet, let alone stick to it. With the Mediterranean diet, you don't have to worry about any of this. You can feel a bit hungry at first, and you might crave sugar, especially if it was a large part of your previous diet, but those symptoms will subside and pretty soon, you will be on your way to adhering to this new eating regimen.

What Foods Make Up the Base of the Diet?

Unlike with some other diets where the rules are clear and set (sometimes even too strict), with this way of eating you don't have to worry much. There is an abundance of ways to follow the Mediterranean diet. The beauty of this way of eating is the liberty it provides when it comes to food choices. There are guidelines, but they are not as strict as some other diets. Let's list the main foods you will eat if you go Mediterranean:

1. Fruits and vegetables

   You can't imagine a Mediterranean meal without vegetables, and if you see someone from the Mediterranean snacking, it is probably on fruit. Fruits and vegetables might be the main reason this diet works so well. Not only are they rich in fiber and therefor satiating and gut-friendly, they also carry a plethora of vitamins and minerals.

   You should stock up on leafy greens that will be the base for most of your salads. There is lettuce, spinach, arugula, and watercress, and you can also try corn salad and Chinese cabbage.

For fruit and other vegetables, you can't go wrong, as long as it is fresh and has no added sugar. There is no fruit that is less Mediterranean than another. However, people in the Mediterranean usually eat seasonal fruit and vegetables, so you might want to consider that if you are someone who craves tomato in December and ends up eating something that vaguely resembles a tomato at a huge price. Not only are seasonal fruits and vegetables more budget friendly, they are usually healthier, tastier and easier to find.

2. Grains and legumes

I combined these into one category because they work best when together. Combining grains and legumes will in most cases give us a complete protein (containing all or most of the nine essential amino acids). We all need protein to gain muscle and lose weight the right way.

Most people rely on meat, eggs and dairy for their main protein sources. However, people from the Mediterranean found that it's best to limit their meat intake and opt for grains and legumes instead.

Nowadays you can choose from a myriad of grains, but some of the most popular are:

- Oats – a cheap and healthy option for a healthy gut, rich in protein and antioxidants. (Whenever you can, make your own oatmeal, instead of eating the pre-made ones, as they tend to be much higher in sugar). Oats can taste great with both sweet and savory foods added.

- Quinoa – not only is quinoa rich in protein, it is also among the most complete plant proteins. It can be expensive in some parts of the world, so feel free to trade it for something else if you are on a tight budget.

- Buckwheat – if you suffer from a gluten intolerance or sensitivity, buckwheat is the way to go. Not only is it gluten free, its protein profile is similar to that of quinoa, making it a powerful tool for building muscle. Buckwheat flour is a great replacement for wheat flour, so be sure to give buckwheat crepes a try.

- Millet – rich in vitamins and higher in healthy fats than other grains, millet is also a clear choice for anybody with respiratory issues, such as asthma, as it doesn't contain the common allergens found in other grains. One interesting way to include millet in your diet is in a soup. Trust me, it's fantastic.

- Barley – as it contains beta-glucan, a simple carb that our body can't digest, barley has long been known to keep insulin from spiking after big meals. Barley tea is popular in Italy, but you can use it in your cooking as well.

Combining grains with legumes can provide you with a complete protein, but it can also be an interesting cooking experience. You can't go wrong with choosing legumes you like, but it's important to change them up a bit once in a while, so you don't end up always eating the same thing. There are so many choices:

- Peas – rich in protein and fiber, peas are as healthy as they are cheap, versatile and tasty. They also promote gut health, especially in elderly people. When buying fresh peas, look for the ones that are colored light green; they are younger and often tastier. Dark green old ones can be chewy and bitter.

- Beans – they are all highly satiating, rich in protein and low in calories. Most of them are cheap, too. So don't scratch your head over choosing the best bean among navy, pinto, black, or plain old kidney beans. Find that ones that are the most affordable, or the ones that you like most. Eventually you can try them all, see what you like, and mix them up every now and then.

- Chickpeas – there is not a big difference between chickpeas and other legumes when it comes to health benefits. They, too, can help lower cholesterol, promote weight loss, and support gut health and insulin sensitivity.

What makes chickpeas special is their texture. They taste quite different from other legumes, and as such they make a great choice for salads, or when you get tired of eating the same thing over and over again.

If you want a healthy spread and are growing tired of peanut butter, give hummus a try. You can make it on your own or buy some in the whole foods store.

- Lentils – One cup of lentils contains 90% of your daily vitamin B9 requirements. This vitamin plays a crucial role in turning food into energy (it helps us convert carbohydrates into glucose that our body can use as fuel) and keeping our insulin levels in check. This makes them a useful tool for weight management. They are tasty and can be cooked in various ways, so you won't get tired of them so easily.

3. Nuts and seeds

Nuts and seeds are a staple food in many diets, due to their high protein and healthy fat content. Almonds, walnuts, cashews, sunflower seeds, pumpkin seeds, chia seeds and Brazil nuts all make excellent allies in the fight for brain health and longevity.

Not only are they rich in antioxidants and fiber, they are also rich in vitamins and minerals that most of us lack. For a long time, nuts and seeds had a bad rep due to the misconception that fats make you fat. Now that we know caloric surplus is what makes us gain weight, healthy fats are back in the game. It's always a bad idea to exclude an entire food group from your diet, and fats have been banished for far too long. Fats are important for our general health, but especially our heart, brain and eyesight.

However, fats are more calorie expensive (yes, even the good kind). As we established earlier, in comparison to 4Kcal per gram for protein and carbs, a gram of fat holds 9Kcal. Even though there is no mechanism that changes nuts to belly fat immediately, we have to be aware of the fact that it can be easy to overeat on nuts and seeds.

4. Olive oil, herbs and spices

Olive oil can fit into the previous category as it is another source of healthy fats, but it deserves a place of its own, due to its popularity and prevalence in this diet. Indeed, it is difficult to imagine a single Mediterranean dish that doesn't include olive oil.

Oleic acid, the largest part (3/4) of olive oil has many proven health benefits, most famously, reducing inflammation and decreasing the risk of cancer (it has beneficial effects on genes linked to cancer, and a high amount of antioxidants). Additionally, olive oil can promote brain health and improve cognitive function, and it has antibacterial properties.

Herbs and spices are in this category because they go hand in hand with olive oil. Also, they are part of the reason the Mediterranean diet is so healthy. One thing we don't lack in this day and age is sodium. Yes, we need it, but not nearly as much as we tend to consume. Replacing salt with spices and herbs can make a big difference, not only from curbing the amount of sodium we consume, but also because of the health benefits of herbs and spices such as basil, parsley, sage, saffron, rosemary, thyme and oregano.

5. Fish and seafood

Fish and seafood are an amazing source of complete protein that comes cheap calorie wise. They are also a rich source of healthy fatty acids, most notably omega-3s. Depending on where you live, some fish may be easier or more difficult to find, but remember to include both white fish (richer in protein) and red fish (richer in healthy fats) in your diet.

It's difficult to say how much of a good thing is too much, and the main reason for caution when it comes to seafood is the possibility of mercury poisoning. For most people this is not a problem, but it can be dangerous for pregnant women or women who are breastfeeding, as well as for the children. The rule of thumb is: try to eat seafood at least twice a week, and try to limit fish that is highest in mercury (tuna, halibut, shark, swordfish, etc.).

Another thing to look out for is allergies and food sensitivities. Some people react to seafood strongly, and their stomachs give them hell after a meal. This doesn't necessarily mean that there was something wrong with the shrimp or that the squid has gone bad. It's more likely that you lack the enzymes needed to digest certain types of seafood. What's worse is that you can be totally fine eating clams, and then experience stomach discomfort after eating oysters. Go easy on yourself and figure out what works best for you. If you are trying something for the first time, trust me, try it at home.

6. Eggs and dairy

Eggs and dairy are not forbidden in the Mediterranean diet, but they are to be eaten in moderation. I am not saying eggs and dairy are bad for you, but people on the Mediterranean diet curb them because their fat requirements are already met through olive oil, oily fish, seafood, avocado, seeds and nuts.

However, you can still eat them from time to time. Eggs are versatile, affordable, and a complete protein.

Milk is another thing we try to consume in smaller quantities when following this diet, but there are some milk products that are quite common in the Mediterranean diet, such as Greek yoghurt, kefir and fresh cheese.

7. Red meat and red wine

People from the Mediterranean have never eaten much pork or beef. This might be because they did not have much cattle, or because bovines were more useful working in the field than as food (the terrain was pretty unforgiving), but regardless of the reason, people ate less meat from pigs, cows and goats.

For this reason, people from the Mediterranean have a much lower risk of developing diabetes or cardiovascular diseases. Red meat contains saturated fats and is high in calories, especially when compared to seafood, fish and legumes.

Before you ditch the red meat altogether, it is not all bad. Red meat is higher in creatine than other meats, and it contains minerals that are otherwise difficult to consume in large quantities. Just keep your consumption moderate.

Red wine is pretty much the same deal. It is not inherently bad, but people tend to misuse it too often for doctors to recommend it in good conscience. It is understandable why people think that wine is an irreplaceable part of the Mediterranean diet. After all, almost every movie or picture showcasing this part of the world has somebody reaching for a bottle of good old red.

Like with most things, the takeaway with red wine is not that alcohol is bad in and of itself, but rather that you should limit the amount you consume if you want to reap the benefits without the adverse effects. The general guideline is to keep your alcohol consumption under 14 units per week.

8. Poultry

Poultry, such as chicken and turkey, is not a huge part of the Mediterranean diet. This doesn't mean that you can't have chicken at all; you can eat more of it than red meat. It's lower in calories and unhealthy fats, and is a good source of protein with a high biological value.

Given that the meat industry is not the most responsible (especially in developing countries where laws are less rigid and regulations are not followed as closely), I always encourage people to find cage-free, organic, grass-fed chicken or turkey.

Example Shopping List - For the Week

If you fail to plan, you are planning to fail. I know it's cliché, but no truer words have been said about diet adherence. I highly advise thinking ahead and being careful if you are trying to make a new habit, especially if the change is not easy or pleasant. If you currently have a sedentary lifestyle, it's not going to be easy to maintain motivation to exercise every day. Sticking to the diet plan might be even more challenging.

Knowing that you must do something is one thing but putting it into practice can be overwhelming if you dive too deep too fast. To help you start off on the right foot, here is how you can organize your shopping for the week. Feel free to change anything that doesn't work for you, and keep in mind that there are many other ways to go about it.

You should start by easing into it and keeping things simple. To do that, you can divide your food into categories by macronutrients:

- Protein

    - Getting protein in bulk can be cumbersome. However, it's easier if you purchase a week's worth of food at a time. It's ideal to buy fresh seafood or fish every morning, but we don't all live by the sea, nor do we all have time to roam the fish market every morning. Do the next best thing. Buy frozen seafood and fish at your nearest grocery store.

      In the beginning it's enough to buy three servings of fish (be sure to rotate between white and oily now and then, and opt for the fish with lower mercury content) and two servings of seafood. To top things off, buy two servings of chicken breast. Your seven big meals (it can be your lunch or dinner, depending on your schedule) are on their way.

- Carbohydrates

  - We are going to divide carbs into three subcategories: grains, legumes and vegetables.

    Grains are the simplest to find and the easiest to buy. Besides quinoa or millet in some parts of the world, they are among the most affordable foods. Not only that, but you can also buy them in bulk and be done with it due to their long shelf life. If you can afford experimenting with your grains, see what works best for you. Depending on your choice, your options for the first week are:

    - Buy a pouch of couscous and brown rice

    - Buy a pack of rice, quinoa, millet and oats

    Legumes are as affordable as grains. How they differ is the time needed to prepare them. Just imagine cooking rice, and now replace rice with navy beans. If you don't have the time to soak them in water overnight, your cooking could take up a huge chunk of your day. That's where buying canned beans, peas, string beans and lentils comes into play. I know it is not perfect, but it still beats fast food and other unhealthy options. You never know when your schedule will free up and you will have more time on your hands.

The weekly recommendation is purchasing seven cans of legumes of your choosing. If possible, try to mix them up and buy as many different kinds as you can. If you have the time, you can also purchase some raw beans, lentils, chickpeas or peas, depending on your taste or their availability.

You can munch on vegetables as much as you like when following almost any diet and the Mediterranean diet is no different. Purchasing them fresh is best, especially when it comes to the leafy greens that will be the staple food for most of your salads. To keep your food expenses from skyrocketing, try to buy seasonal vegetables and buy them a day at a time.

Of course, not everyone can eat this way for various reasons, such as lack of free time for shopping and low income. However, you have some options regardless of the circumstances. If there are no fresh vegetables in your store, you can buy frozen and it still beats eating French fries. For those of you who lack the time to prepare food, opt for prewashed and chopped vegetables.

For one week, you can either buy fresh veggies every day or buy frozen ones, but you should have at least 14 servings of vegetables per week, as you can't really overeat on them. Try not to get stuck in a rut with eating the same thing over and over again.

Recently websites and magazines have been aggrandizing certain foods (vegetables and grains especially). They write embellished articles about "super foods," or a miraculous berry, or a secret that big pharma doesn't want you to know. In these articles, the positive effects of fruits and vegetables are blown out of proportion with an abundance of false claims. There is no such a thing as a super food. Just try to eat a wide variety of vegetables to get a full profile of vitamins and minerals (and not get bored in the process).

- Fats

  – Fats are the easiest macronutrient to find on the Mediterranean diet because most of your choices are already made. You can mix avocado and nuts and the rest will be taken care of by oily fish and olive oil.

    Be sure to choose extra virgin olive oil instead of its refined counterpart. Even though the difference in the price can be mind-boggling, trust me, it is more than worth it.

    Refined olive oil has been treated with solvents to mask the odors that aren't there in the first place with extra virgin olive oil. Usually, those smells come from olives that were past their expiration date. They lack the omega-3s, antioxidants and polyphenols that are present in extra virgin olive oil, which contains nothing but oil squeezed from olives.

    Avocado has a longer shelf life than other vegetables due to its higher fat content, so you can buy a pack if you find a budget-friendly offer.

    Nuts are not only cheap but available year-round thanks to their long shelf life. You can't go wrong with them, so try every nut you can find and figure out which ones you like. They complement both savory and sweet dishes alike, and roasting them or blanching them gives them a whole new texture and taste. So even if you only like hazelnuts, there are still at least three different ways to prepare them.

The weekly recommendation is: a handful of nuts for every day (the choice is yours), three avocados, and around 250cc of olive oil.

- Spices, herbs and dressings
  - You can use a huge variety of spices and herbs and not go wrong. If you are on a tight budget, you can use the things you have in your house. If you want to experiment, give some of these a try: basil, thyme, rosemary, oregano, curry, parsley, sage, and don't forget ground pepper.

    As for dressings, I wouldn't complicate things too much from the get-go. Use primarily olive oil and balsamic vinegar, but later down the road, you can experiment with Greek yogurt, lemon, honey, basil and parsley dressings. We will talk more about that in the recipes section.

    The takeaway message is to go with what you like at first and try to incorporate new spices after a while to get a fuller picture of what the Mediterranean really tastes like.

When you put it all together, an example shopping list for the week could look something like this:

- 16oz of cod
- 2 medium size chicken breasts

- 10oz of shrimp

- ½lb of couscous

- ½lb of brown rice

- 4 cans of beans (white, red, navy and pinto)

- 1 can of lentils

- 1 can of chickpeas

- 1 can of peas

- 2 cups of broccoli

- 2 cups of cauliflower

- 2 cups of bell peppers

- 2 cups of lettuce

- 4 large tomatoes

- 2 cups of spinach

- 2oz of hazelnuts

- 2oz of almonds

- 2oz of cashews

- 2oz of walnuts

- 3 avocados

- 250cc of olive oil

Example Weekly Meal Plan

The Mediterranean diet is mainly about what foods you eat and not necessarily when or how you eat them, so following this diet does not collide with any specific eating schedule. You can combine the Mediterranean diet and intermittent fasting or any other eating protocol that works for you.

I wouldn't recommend too long of a fasting period right off the bat. You should give your body enough time to adapt to calorie restriction. Later, if you want, you can introduce intermittent fasting.

To make matters simple, let's assume you have an average daily eating schedule: three meals and a snack. This works for most people. It's enough to help minimize snacking and avoid feeling hungry, unfocused, and low on energy. Also, this meal frequency (especially with enough protein per meal – over 20 grams) promotes protein synthesis and helps you build muscle which leads to faster and steadier fat loss in the long run. To paint a clearer picture, this is what a typical meal plan would look like on a week of the Mediterranean diet. Don't worry if you're confused about some of the recipes' names; we will explain them in the following chapters.

Monday

Breakfast: Whole wheat toast with rubbed-on garlic, drizzled with olive oil

Lunch: Quinoa salad with zucchini, dried tomatoes and baby carrots

Snack: A handful of walnuts and an apple

Dinner: Grilled salmon with vegetables

Tuesday

Breakfast: Greek yogurt with berries, honey and crunched almonds

Lunch: Seafood and tomato sauce risotto

Snack: Strawberries

Dinner: Grilled chicken breast and avocado slices seasoned with lemon and pepper

Wednesday

Breakfast: Boiled eggs, a slice of toast and some brie

Lunch: Tuna salad with couscous, eggplant, lettuce, broccoli and crunched peanuts

Snack: Orange juice and a handful of cashews

Dinner: A salad topped with hummus, beans and blanched carrots

Thursday

Breakfast: Whole wheat toast with ricotta cheese

Lunch: Shrimp salad with lettuce, avocado, cucumber, lentils and Dijon mustard

Snack: Dried fruit

Dinner: White fish with asparagus, carrots and tomatoes

Friday

Breakfast: Fruit of your choice with fresh cheese or yogurt

Lunch: Mackerel with sweet potato and olives

Snack: Handful of roasted hazelnuts

Dinner: Veggie salad with lettuce, chickpeas, beans, lentils, blanched broccoli and carrots, dressed with balsamic vinegar and olive oil

Saturday

Breakfast: Omelet with tomatoes and fresh herbs with a side of feta cheese

Lunch: Mushroom potage with chicken breast cubes and croutons

Snack: Greek yogurt with berries

Dinner: Grilled seafood with vegetables and iceberg salad

Sunday

Breakfast: whole wheat sandwich with fresh cheese, tomatoes and hummus

Lunch: Grilled white fish with lemon avocado salad and arugula

Snack: Berries and a handful of nuts

Dinner: Quinoa bowl with shrimp, peppers, mushrooms and cherry tomatoes

As I said, this is just an example of what a week of eating could look like. If you want to eat all your food in two sittings each day, do that. If you want to follow a once-a-day eating protocol, I won't stop you. And now that we are equipped with the knowhow, let's get a bit more specific with the recipes.

Recipes

Food itself is the most fun part of this whole endeavor, and it is as delicious as it is healthy. Keep in mind that all the recipes here make one serving, so you will need to multiply the quantity of ingredients by the number of people you are cooking for.

Feel free to change any part of the recipes so they make more sense for you, be it for the sake of taste or food sensitivities. Don't worry if not everything turns out to look or taste how you expected. One of the healthiest characteristics of the Mediterranean way of life is low stress levels, so don't ruin all your hard work by worrying too much.

A Word of Caution

Losing weight is determined by caloric deficit, like we have previously stated. Regardless of how healthy you eat, expending more calories than you consume will always be a requirement for weight loss. Be sure to keep that in mind when starting this diet.

Also, the numbers given in the chapter that follows are just guidelines. Everybody's needs are different, so be sure to check your calorie requirements (you can use a TDEE calculator online if you don't have access to a more precise apparatus) and adjust the portions accordingly.

Before we begin, there is another thing we must clarify. Weight loss isn't everything. Most people reading this just want to see the scale numbers go down, and fast. That can be detrimental to your long-term success for a couple of reasons.

First, even if you don't see the numbers going down, that doesn't mean that no progress is being made. Your body can undergo an unbelievable transformation without dropping a pound in weight. If you start exercising at the same time that you start this diet, you might experience a decrease in body fat and an increase in muscle mass. Two people who weigh 200 pounds can look drastically if one is more muscular than the other.

If you are focused solely on losing weight as fast as possible, you might be doing more harm than good. Losing a lot of weight in a short period of time can result in muscle wasting and a slowing of metabolism. Rapid weight loss should not be achieved at the expense of muscle mass. Otherwise, your weight will bounce back as quickly as you can say, "yo-yo effect."

This means that even if you manage to reach your goal weight, it will be difficult to maintain it without enough muscle as the most active tissue, metabolically speaking. To minimize muscle wasting, you can do physical exercise (especially resistance training) and include plenty of protein in your diet.

The message to take home from this is that Rome wasn't built in a day. Try to set realistic goals and be patient enough to see the results. Give yourself enough time to see them the right way, and at the right tempo.

Breakfast Recipes

Salmon, Eggs and Avocado Toast

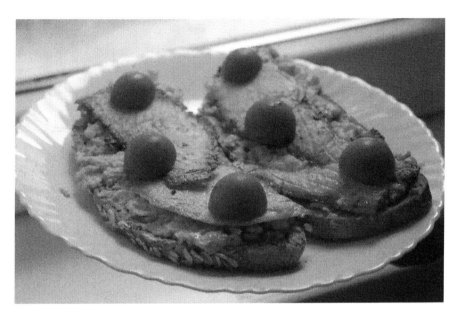

Salmon was once discarded as the fish with the most calories, and avoided even by bodybuilders who need the most calories to meet their goals. Since the era of fat avoidance has ended, salmon has experienced its renaissance.

If you want to supply your brain and body with the energy they need, this breakfast option will work wonders. Once you grasp the preparation process, it's easy to make. It doesn't take me longer than 20 minutes. Also, since most us have limited time in the morning, it's great news that you can get everything you need for breakfast in just six or seven bites. Don't be fooled by the small quantity; this meal will not leave you high and dry and reaching for snacks in a half hour. Thanks to its high fat content and complex carbohydrates, you will feel full well into the afternoon.

Ingredients:

- 80g of raw salmon

- 2 slices of whole wheat toast

- 2 eggs

- ½ avocado

- 1tbsp of organic butter or olive oil

- 1tbsp of lemon juice

- 4 cherry tomatoes

- Herbs and spices to your liking (I like oregano and garlic)

Preparation:

- Slice the avocado and mash it with a fork (ripe avocado will make the job easier). Add some freshly squeezed lemon juice and black pepper.

- Chop up a clove or two of garlic and sauté with olive oil or butter over low to medium heat. Add eggs that you have previously whisked with a bit of Himalayan salt and pepper. Scramble to your liking but try not to leave them too runny so they don't drip from the toast.

- Fry the salmon in a drip of olive oil. For sushi lovers, keep in mind that salmon can be left raw as well. Just be sure to cut it into thin slices.

- Toast the bread and spread the avocado mash. Then add the eggs and salmon and top it all off with herbs and spices.

Morning Pizza

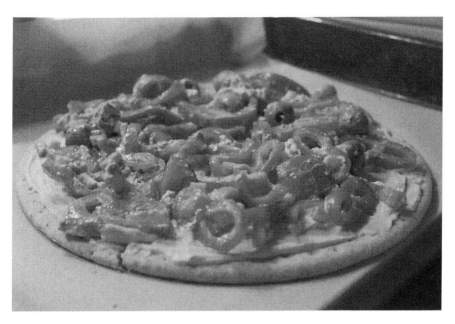

I know I said that pizza is not a part of the Mediterranean diet, but bear with me. Not only is this meal healthy and delicious, it also requires very little time and no cooking at all. The combination of slow digesting carbs from the crust and hummus and the fiber from the vegetables makes this a satiating and gut-friendly meal.

What makes this a great breakfast choice is that it can be changed to fit anyone's needs and tastes. You can choose the combo of vegetables that you like and change it up every now and then, so it's almost impossible for this dish to get old for anyone with a bit of imagination.

Ingredients:

- Whole wheat pizza crust - premade or from the store (if you don't have the time to make the pizza crust, this can just as easily be a morning burrito with whole wheat tortillas)

- 50g of feta cheese (tofu also works if you want to avoid dairy)

- A cup of chopped vegetables of your choice (try to include something crunchy for the sake of texture)

- 4tbsp of hummus (if you have some time on your hands, it's easy to make your own)

- 1tbsp of balsamic vinegar

Preparation:

- Chop the vegetables and put them in a bowl. Mix them up with the feta cheese and balsamic vinegar.

- Spread the hummus over the pizza crust or tortilla. You can use more hummus for a richer taste.

- If you want to make it more exciting, you can top it with fresh arugula and crunched peanuts.

Lunch Recipes

Seafood Tomato Sauce Risotto

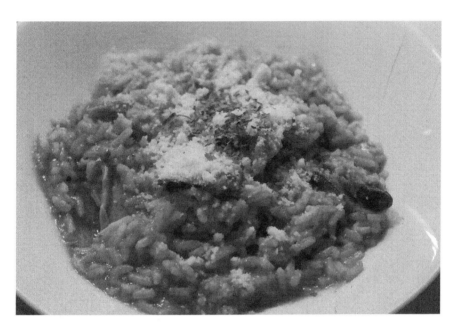

Seafood risotto can be a great choice for dinner or lunch. This is a healthy meal that doesn't take long to make. If you are in a hurry and need to make something fast, but still impress your guest(s) with your cooking skills, give this a chance.

This is a one-pan dish, so you don't have to worry about piles of dishes in your kitchen. Also, it doesn't have to cost too much and it won't leave you hungry. All of this makes this dish a great choice for students who want to live healthier on a budget.

Ingredients:

- Canned tomato sauce (or freshly made if you have time)

- 250g of raw seafood

- One small onion

- 60g of uncooked rice

- 20g of grated Parmesan cheese (optional)

- Chopped parsley and basil

- 1tbsp of olive oil

- Pepper

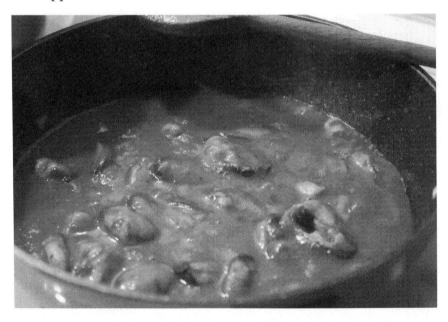

Preparation:

- Chop up onions and put them in a pan with some water, pepper and three drops of olive oil. Once the onions are soft and transparent, add the seafood.

- Once the water almost evaporates, pour the tomato sauce and cook on low heat for 20 minutes. Be sure to stay close to the cooker so you can stir as the tomato sauce boils quickly compared to water.

- In the rice cooker or a different bowl, cook rice to your liking.

- Pour a tablespoon of olive oil and mix in the rice with the seafood and tomato sauce. Let it cook for 5 more minutes, while stirring, until it thickens.

- Remove from heat, add grated parmesan and season with parsley and basil.

Quinoa Chicken Bowl

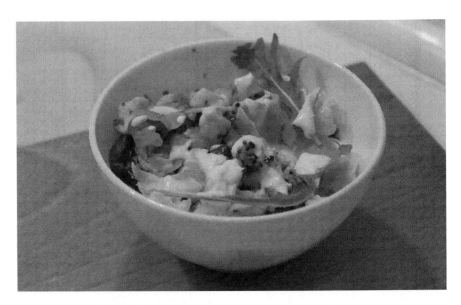

Quinoa is not your typical Mediterranean plant, as it originates from South America. However, its high protein content and other health benefits make it an irreplaceable part of the Mediterranean diet if you enjoy its taste.

Chicken breast is known for its short cooking time (if you cut it thin enough, 7-8 minutes per side will more than suffice, and if you cut it like we will here, you will end up with even less cooking). Quinoa is pretty much the same, as it requires much less cooking time than rice or other grains (couscous is the champion).

Ingredients:

For the dish:

- ½ cup of quinoa

- 150g of chicken breast (cage free if possible)

- ½ cup of red beans (or any other beans of your liking)

- 1 tbsp of olive oil

- ¼ cup of corn

- ½ avocado

- ½ cup of lettuce

- Arugula, pepper, basil and garlic

For the dressing:

- 1 lemon

- 2 cloves of garlic

- White wine vinegar (optional)

- ½ cup of plain Greek yogurt

- 1tsp of sugar

- 1tsp of salt

- Extra virgin olive oil

Preparation:

- Slice the chicken breast into thin slices and marinade with olive oil, pepper and garlic. You can skillet-fry it or grill it depending on your preference.

- Rinse the quinoa with cold water and place in a small pot. Add in a double amount of water and bring it to a boil. Let it simmer until the quinoa absorbs the water and the rest of it evaporates. This and the previous step can be done ahead of time, if you want to have a cold dish on a hot day.

- Chop the lettuce and arugula and add it to the quinoa together with corn and beans. Add some basil and ground garlic and mix it all up.

- Slice the avocado and arrange it on the top of the salad bowl with the chicken.

- Mash the garlic and whisk it together with the Greek yogurt, white wine vinegar, olive oil, sugar, salt and 2tbsp of freshly squeezed lemon juice.

Side Dish Recipes

Bean Salad

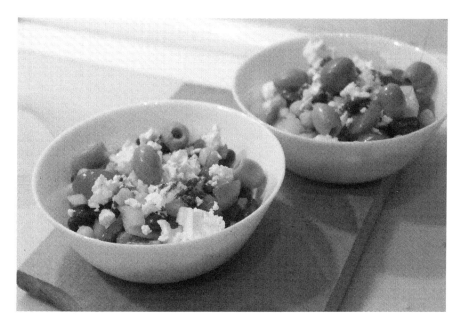

Surely there is no way to make a satisfying meal in under ten minutes with no cooking, right? Think again. Not only can it be done, but this meal can tick most of the boxes in the healthy food checklist. If you are looking for a quick dish that doesn't require ninja-level mastery in the kitchen, this is it.

I listed this salad as a side dish because it's one of my favorites but make no mistake – this meal can work as a lunch, dinner or breakfast. It contains enough carbs to provide you with enough energy to tackle your day. It is also rich in vitamins, minerals, healthy fats and fiber, which are all necessary to make you feel energized and motivated.

Another great trait of this salad is that it can last for a few days if you seal it properly and keep it in the refrigerator.

Ingredients:

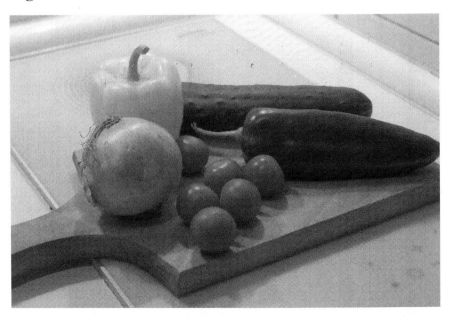

- ½ cup of beans of your choice (chickpeas can work as well; make sure you rinse them well to avoid the "canned taste" if you are not cooking them yourself)

- ½ cup of cherry tomatoes (or regular tomatoes cut into cubes)

- A small cucumber (sliced into circles or half-circles depending on the size)

- ½ of a small onion, sliced or chopped (red works best, but it's not set in stone)

- 1 bell pepper, chopped

- 8-10 olives of your choice

- 1 small sweet pointed pepper (sliced into rings)

- Basil leaves (three to four will suffice)

- A handful of crumbled feta cheese

Dressing:

- 2 tbsp olive oil

- 2 tbsp balsamic vinegar

- Ground garlic (a teaspoon or more, depending on how fond of garlic you are)

- Salt, pepper and herbs (oregano, parsley and sage work for me, but feel free to experiment)

Preparation:

- Rinse the beans well if they're canned.

- Cut, chop and slice the vegetables.

- Mix the ingredients for the dressing together and check it to see if you like the taste, then set it aside.

- Put the beans in a large bowl and add the rest of the ingredients except for the cheese. I like to first drizzle the dressing and then add in the cheese so it remains as salty as it's made, but don't bother yourself with that if you don't care about the taste of feta cheese itself.

- Enjoy as either a side dish or as the main course if you are in a rush.

Dinner Recipes

Chicken Spinach Soup

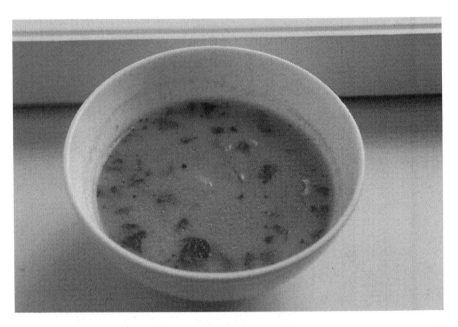

If you don't think soup counts as dinner, you are not alone; I use to think the same. Where I come from, soup is usually eaten before a meal to warm up your stomach. If it's hot outside, you skip the soup, simple as that. That a soup can be a full meal came as quite a revelation to me.

It was much later when I discovered how refreshing and nourishing soups and potages can be. It was then when I started experimenting and trying out different recipes like this. It may not be my all-time favorite (I don't really have one), but this soup is my savior on hot summer nights when I don't feel like cooking for too long.

This soup works well cold and hot alike. I like to eat it for dinner because it keeps you full and away from midnight snacking without being too heavy and difficult to digest like some of the oilier meals.

It's easy to find most of these ingredients, but like always, feel free to change anything or make it easier for yourself (for example, by buying premade pesto if you don't want to make it).

Ingredients:

- 3 tbsp olive oil

- 2 small carrots, chopped

- 150g chicken breast, cut into cubes

- 3 cups of chicken broth

- Garlic, minced

- A handful of baby spinach, chopped

- ¼ cup of kidney beans

- 3 tbsp grated parmesan

- Basil leaves (a handful)

- Ground pepper and herbs and spices to taste (oregano, thyme and marjoram all work)

Preparation:

- Dice the chicken into bite-sized cubes. You can do this before cooking or just after cooking and just before adding in the beans and the spinach in step 4.

- Heat up 2 tablespoons of olive oil and add the carrots and chicken. Stir them together for around 5 minutes, depending on the heat, but the chicken should be getting brownish towards the end of the process. Add the garlic and stir for a minute or two more.

- Pour in the broth and seasonings and stir well. Bring it all to a boil and then reduce the heat, letting it simmer until the chicken is cooked all the way through. This doesn't usually take long - another five to ten minutes will more than suffice.

- Add the beans and the spinach and bring to a boil again. Be sure to do it carefully and gently, otherwise the spinach will end up a bit mushy and mealy.

- Combine the parmesan, basil and the rest of the olive oil (1 tablespoon is enough) and mix them up in a blender or a food processor. Process until the pesto forms.

- Mix the pesto into the pot and heat until hot. As I already stated, you can serve this dish cold, and the taste is not any worse for it. Enjoy.

Dessert Recipes

Mediterranean Chocolate Cake

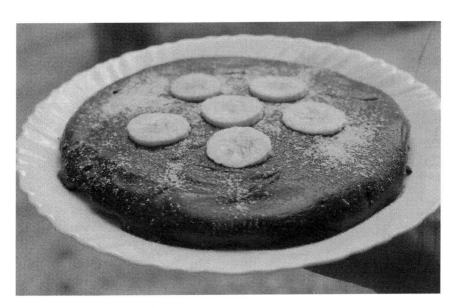

Who says there is no way to enjoy the Mediterranean diet with a sweet tooth? There are many ways to incorporate sweets and still reap the benefits of the Mediterranean diet. With this diet, we try to avoid butter and rely on olive oil as a substitute. I know that doesn't sound quite as yummy, but just give it a try. That way we cut down on the intake of saturated fats in favor of the healthier unsaturated fats that come from olive oil.

Additionally, we can swap refined sugar with something a little healthier, such as fructose from fruit. Not only is fructose less detrimental to our health, but with fruit, we get a nice side dish of fiber, vitamins and minerals. It's not that chocolate cake equals obesity, but there is a way to make it a smidge healthier without compromising the taste.

Ingredients:

For the cake:

- ¾ cup of gluten free flour (buckwheat flour and whole grain work just as well)

- A pinch of baking soda and cinnamon

- ½ cup of cocoa powder

- ½ cup olive oil

- 1 tsp of stevia (or 1 cup of brown or granulated sugar if you are dead set on getting your sugary fix)

- 4 eggs

For the glaze:

- 1 tsp of stevia extract (liquid or powdered) or 1 cup of sugar

- 4 tbsp cocoa powder

- 1 tbsp olive oil

- Pinch of salt

Preparation:

For the cake:

- Preheat the oven to 350⁰F and lay the parchment on a round cake pan.

- Grease it with olive oil.

- Combine the flour, baking soda, cocoa powder and cinnamon in a small pot or bowl.

- In a bigger bowl, whisk the eggs together with salt.

- Add in the sugar or stevia and then pour the contents of the smaller bowl into the big one.

- Mix until smooth while adding the remaining olive oil.

- Bake for around half an hour and then leave it to cool for 15 minutes.

For the glaze:

- In a smaller pot combine water and sugar or stevia until smooth.

- Add in the cocoa and blend well (if you use stevia, you can blend all of this at once; granulated sugar needs a bit more time due to the sheer volume).

- Mix the olive oil and salt.

- Warm the glaze on low heat while stirring non-stop, and be careful not to overheat it (just warm to the touch will do).

- Drizzle the glaze over the cake and enjoy.

Snack Ideas

As you already know, people in the Mediterranean are not huge on snacking. If you want to follow the Mediterranean diet, a simple piece of fruit will do, as will some yogurt or some nuts. But in order to make things a bit more interesting, let's make a snack that combines the best of those three. I give you:

Honey-Topped Yogurt with Fresh Blueberries and Peanuts

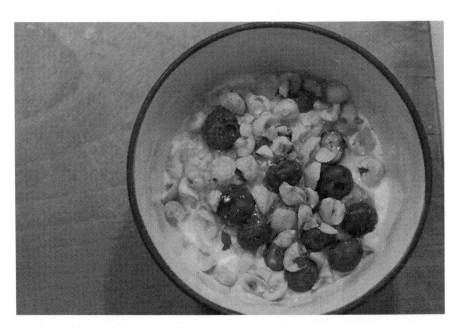

This is more of a pattern than a recipe, as you can change every one of these four ingredients to something similar that is more available, affordable, or simply more to your liking. Put simply, you need something sweet, something crunchy, something yogurt-like and some fruit.

The ratio between them is also just a guideline and will mostly depend on your preferences. However, be careful not to go overboard with the nuts as they are unforgiving calorie-wise.

It goes without saying that it takes almost no time to make this snack and you can easily pack it and take it with you to work or the gym. It works well as a post-workout meal, restoring your glycogen and providing enough protein to promote muscle growth. Also, it doesn't require any special equipment like blenders, food processors or slow cookers.

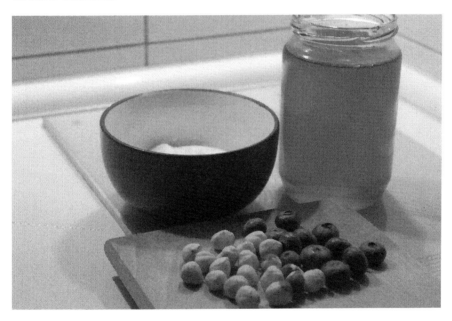

Ingredients:

- A handful of peanuts (or cashews, brazil nuts, walnuts, hazelnuts, almonds, etc.)

- ¾ cup of strawberries (almost any fruit will work, but I recommend using something organic, seasonal, and sweet as Greek yogurt and ricotta already taste a bit sour).

- ½ cup of Greek yogurt (you can replace this with ricotta that is a bit more sour. Cottage cheese is a good choice for athletes because it has the highest protein content of all dairy products. If you are lactose intolerant or vegan, you can use silken tofu).

- 1 tbsp of honey or another sweetener (you can skip the sweetener if the fruit is sweet enough).

Preparation:

- Chop up the fruit first, and then crush the nuts using the dull side of the knife.

- Place the yogurt next to it or mix it all up if you prefer it that way.

- Top it with honey.

- Put it in the freezer and take it with you, especially if you have a busy week ahead.

Conclusion

There is a plethora of ways in which you can organize your diet. Someone who says that there is only one way to do it right is lying, trying to sell you something or both. When thinking about diets and pondering whether a certain eating protocol is right for you, you should weigh all the pros and cons. If its downsides make it impossible or too difficult for you to follow, then that diet is not the best option for you, especially if they outweigh the positive aspects. It doesn't mean that the diet itself is bad, just that it may not be the perfect choice for you.

Pros of the Mediterranean diet:

1. It's easy to understand and follow.

    Once the fog clears about what the Mediterranean diet is and isn't, there is not much left to the imagination. You should eat no junk food, have a lot of vegetables and fruit, opt for complex rather than simple carbs, limit intake of poultry, eggs, dairy and especially red meat, and eat fish and seafood instead. Also, consume healthy fats like olive oil, avocado and nuts.

    There are no strict time schedules, no complicated rules and metrics, and no worrying about every little detail. Thanks to the high fiber intake, it's easy to adhere to this diet as it won't make you feel famished when achieving a caloric deficit.

    Also, it doesn't eliminate or drastically limit any of the macronutrients (fats, carbohydrates or protein), so you have a wide maneuvering space for meeting your daily goals and eating the foods you like in the process.

2. It's healthy.

   You shouldn't fall for marketing schemes that claim miraculous effects of any one food or diet, but there is actual peer-reviewed data supporting the claim that following the Mediterranean diet can be beneficial for your health.

   Nobody can guarantee you longevity, and nobody is risk-free of diseases or ugly conditions that might pop up, but at least this way we have done everything in our power to diminish the risks of that happening, and improve our chances of leading a long and healthy life.

3. It'll help you lose weight.

   We have already said that there are no miracles when it comes to dieting and being fit. Everything requires work and willpower, and the Mediterranean diet can only make your efforts easier by making you feel full longer and supporting your hard work with enough protein to make your body strong and more resistant to putting on weight.

   Also, staying healthy will make you more consistent with your workouts, which in turn makes it even easier to lose weight. It is a virtuous circle where one good thing brings another.

4. It's compatible with various eating patterns and schedules.

   Eating Mediterranean food doesn't get in the way of any specific eating schedule (timewise). This means that you can eat this way and still be able to intermittently fast, for example.

Also, it allows for a greater food choice than some other diets, so regardless of your preferences or allergies, there is always something you can eat that will keep you full.

Some data shows that a higher fat content correlates with people giving food higher ratings, so if the meals contains fats (and with this diet, they usually do), people are more likely to enjoy it.

Cons of the Mediterranean diet:

5. It's difficult to follow if you have certain food allergies.

Food sensitivities usually don't get in the way of this diet as it is unlikely for someone to be allergic to all fruits and vegetables. This diet doesn't eliminate any major food groups so you have plenty of backups even if you can't have some foods for whatever reason.

One allergy that can make matters a little more complicated is an allergy to seafood, but even in that case you needn't despair. Allergies usually don't include the entire food group, so be sure to test which kinds of seafood you are allergic to.

Even if you can't have any of it, there is always something you can do. You can swap it for fish, or eat more vegetables, grains and legumes. You can even swap the seafood for chicken and increase the amount of healthy fats attained from other sources. It's not perfect, but it's better than eating junk food.

6. Some of the foods can seem expensive at first.

Opponents of the Mediterranean diet often bring this up, and it can be true to a point. Some of the food (especially nuts, seafood and avocados) can be pricy in some parts of the world.

For some that seems discouraging, but that's just one of the traps you can fall into before giving it a try. I often hear that eating fish will leave you hungry in less than an hour. Combine that with the fact that in this part of the world, fish is more expensive than pork, and you can understand people's objections.

However, before you decided to go on the Mediterranean diet, you were probably eating way more than you need. Give your appetite a chance to adapt to the new circumstances. What you can do in the meantime to make it easier is eat more vegetables and fruit (you probably weren't eating enough of them before) to keep you full longer and remember that quality trumps quantity of food.

Another way you can save money is by buying in bulk (especially legumes and grains), and buying seasonal fruits and vegetables that are not just cheaper but healthier as well.

Try to Go Full Mediterranean

Yes, following the Mediterranean diet will make an impact on your health and waistline, but it can do so much more if you are willing to go the extra mile. As we have already established, the lifestyle of people from the Mediterranean is a crucial part of their longevity and wellbeing. What I am trying to say is: try to eat and live more like them.

This does not have to be a drastic change and I am by no means trying to tell you that you should sell your house and move to Tuscany. There are ways to incorporate the little things that they do without any radical twists.

For example, walk to the market next time you want to buy a salad. Yes, you can probably buy the same thing in the supermarket down the street (and for less money, probably), but doing things quickly and spending less money just so you have more time to work is not what the Mediterranean way of life is all about.

Start small. Go to the market and talk to the merchants. Maybe you will meet someone new, hear a joke, or see something interesting. No matter what, you will experience something unexpected.

That helps put me in the "now." For that one moment there is no worrying about what will happen at the interview today, or what time the appointment is at the bank, or whether I will have enough time to go to the gym before meeting with colleagues.

You don't need me to tell you this, but the pace at which we are living is way faster than it used to be, and it can be detrimental to us, especially people with a lower threshold for stress and an inability to adapt to change. It is difficult to eliminate all the stressors in our environment, be it a demanding boss, or moving to another city or country, or a complicated period in your relationship.

But we can do something every day to put things in perspective. Yes, you can buy a precooked meal and save yourself some time to work or watch a little TV, but you can also play some music in the background and prepare a healthy meal for yourself. It doesn't have to be a culinary masterpiece; preparing it will be just the change of pace you were looking for.

If you remember to take baby steps and try to move a bit further away from your comfort zone every day, you will soon find out that there is more to life than just work, sleeping and duties. At least to me, the biggest benefit of the Mediterranean diet is that it teaches you how to appreciate the little things and enjoy the moment without overthinking.

You might catch yourself enjoying the cooking and shopping for groceries, and, why not, making dinner for your old and new friends. Amazing things can happen if you are brave enough, and this diet and lifestyle doesn't ask for that much bravery.

If you've enjoyed reading this book, subscribe* to my mailing list for exclusive content and sneak peeks of my future books.

Visit the link below:

http://eepurl.com/gJnw1X

OR

Use the QR Code:

(*Must be 13 years or older to subscribe)

Made in the USA
Columbia, SC
12 June 2020

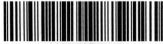
10834721R00043